When Partnering with Your Medical Doctor is Difficult

The Present Day Dilemma in Getting Proper Medical Care

By: James M. Lowrance © 2011

DEDICATION:

To all of my fellow patients seeking compassionate, quality doctors. I offer my sincere wish for you to find a truly-called physician who has your best health care interests at heart and that you will often express your appreciation to them as a partner in your medical diagnoses and treatments.

TABLE OF CONTENTS:

INTRODUCTION:

The health care - medical professionals field, is among the most important callings on earth but doctors and medical workers have very difficult and very stressful jobs. There has also arisen an unmistakable doctor-shortage in many areas of America. This has increased the workload of medical staff and professionals and some of them are experiencing a condition referred to by medical research groups, as "burn out". Doctors can be seriously affected both mentally and physically by this very real and increasing problem. At the same time, medical patients can also be negatively affected, in-fact medical errors are the third leading cause of death in the US currently and the problem has potential to become even worse.

Is there a solution to this problem? As a layperson, non medical professional, I certainly cannot predict either a solution or a worsening of the problem. As a patient with diagnosed medical disorders, I can however express what I believe to be essential actions from both the patient's and doctor's side, that must be taken in order to help us become better-partnered.

It is my sincere hope that whether medical professionals read the chapters that follow or medical patients do, that they will consider these suggestions that are backed by medical research quotes and statistics, with an open mind. The future of our Nation's health care, depends on the actions we take now, to improve and to maintain its quality.

-Jim Lowrance

CHAPTER ONE

Personal Experiences that Inspired my Medical Patient Proactiveness

I will start by relating my first experience with an incorrect diagnosis, which occurred at a cardiologist's office in Texas, when I was in my teens. An MD who was treating a chest cold I developed, informed my parents that he heard a faint indication of a heart murmur in me and recommended a heart specialist for further evaluation. The cardiologist who eventually evaluated the murmur, diagnosed me with "Wolff-Parkinson-White Syndrome" – a serious type of murmur, that in some cases requires surgery to be corrected, to prevent heart failure and ventricular fibrillation (a non life sustaining erratic heart beat) if serious symptoms develop.

Approximately 20 years later, in my late 30s, then living in Oklahoma, I had the heart murmur re-evaluated by another cardiologist, who ruled out my ever having this heart syndrome. He stated that they were mistaken because the condition is lifelong, unless corrected surgically (he specialized in this syndrome).

My disappointment in the earlier diagnosis, was in the fact that I lived with significant anxiety regarding the syndrome, for 20 years and when I experienced any heart palpitations, this often resulted in panic attacks due to my fear of the condition. I often wondered during those years if I might experience cardiac arrest or be required to have open-heart surgery. While the corrected diagnosis was a tremendous relief to me, the anxiety I experienced for many years, negatively affected my quality of life.

In the year 2003, while still living in my current state of Oklahoma at age 40, I was diagnosed with autoimmune thyroid disease, which caused me to become hypothyroid (underactive thyroid gland). Before my diagnosis, I had made several doctor-visits, complaining to them about multiple symptoms that I believed pointed to a medical condition (i.e. severe fatigue, extremely dry skin, hives and mild swelling in my face). Even considering the fact that I was also suffering from bouts of severe anxiety and mild-to-moderate depression, the physical symptoms obviously needed evaluation.

This is especially true with the fact that MANY medical conditions include emotional manifestations as part of their symptom-complexes.

Rather than the doctors I first attended ordering me proper medical testing, to rule-out or to confirm any underlying medical conditions, as a cause of my symptoms, they instead resorted to immediate diagnoses of emotional disorder only and I was offered antidepressants as a treatment for my symptoms. I finally insisted on blood lab testing and my thyroid disease showed up clearly on the results. I had two abnormally low thyroid hormone results, an elevated TSH level (a pituitary hormone that elevates with hypothyroidism) and I was found positive for two thyroid antibodies (killer cells from the immune system that attack the thyroid gland), with the level of one being nearly 500 points above normal.

I was started on treatment for the underactive thyroid, via hormone replacement therapy. As the years went by however I found that I was experiencing widespread body pain and neurological type symptoms.

I began the quest once again, to find out what was causing my unrelieved symptoms, in spite of being treated for my hypothyroidism. I felt certain that another medical condition or possibly more than one was occurring co-morbid to my thyroid disease (together with it).

My first visits to several different doctors, yielded the same type of results as when I sought diagnosis for my thyroid disorder -- they again were recommending prescription antidepressants. I wondered if my wife actually believed me regarding the frequency in which these medications were being recommended and I asked her to go with me to a visit with a new doctor. To her amazement (but not to mine), this doctor again recommended a frequently prescribed Selective Serotonin Reuptake Inhibitor (an SSRI antidepressant).

According to a news release on the CNN Health website, published in year-2007, the Centers for Disease Control reported that antidepressants are the most commonly-prescribed drugs in America, second only to hypertensive medications.

The report also mentions that psychiatrists are happy to see this statistic because it indicates that Americans are now more open to pharmaceutical help for their emotions. The questions arise however, as to how many of these patients request the drugs and how many are give the recommendation by their doctors and whether or not patients were first evaluated for medical conditions or referred to mental health professionals. I again chose to refuse the medication in my case and I scheduled an appointment with yet another new doctor.

The new doctor ordered blood tests but an area of testing not ordered for me that I actually requested from him, were my vitamin levels. I was aware of the fact that some essential vitamins can become low in some people, such as vitamins B12, D and B6, which can cause neurological symptoms. The doctor responded to this request by saying that vitamins aren't really important. He added that it was rare for men to become deficient and that it was usually women who were found to be in need of vitamin replacement therapies for deficiencies. He did however order me testing to rule out diabetes, which had actually been done by previous doctors.

When Partnering with Your Medical Doctor is Difficult

He then suggested I take an antidepressant and this recommendation would be repeated at several succeeding office visits with him (my thyroid hormone therapy required blood retests to be repeated every few months). The suggestion was made due to the unrelieved body aches I continued to experience and although I refused the antidepressants, I remained with this doctor for a period of time.

At this point, I became completely frustrated with doctors and for my unrelieved symptoms; I simply began to take natural supplements to strengthen my adrenal glands and to increase my energy levels. I also took over-the-counter pain medications for the body pain. This actually helped for a period of time however, I began to experience worsening pain symptoms in my arms and legs and my muscle-weakness, which manifested even prior to my being treated for hypothyroidism, was worsening. This problem was eventually revealed as peripheral neuropathy, however, in my case the symptoms developed a bit atypically (not the type of progression usually seen with nerve disease).

As all of this was occurring, I witnessed an alarming number of mistakes being made by medical staff at doctor's offices and hospitals. My first thyroid tests, were lost for several months by the hospital they were performed at but they assured me that the results were normal and not to worry about them. I eventually demanded that they be tracked-down and once receiving them, I found that I had thyroid disease and the results were not in fact "normal".

There were also several occasions in which tests that were ordered, ended-up not being performed, due to doctor's office staff not entering all of the blood test codes on requisition forms or they would enter them incorrectly. I remember two occasions in which this required me to have a second blood draw performed due to failure by them, in adding the correct tests. I actually had to have a hole-punch skin biopsy repeated on my left leg at one point as well (two hole punches each time for a total of four) due to doctor's office staff, entering a wrong code on the requisition form, resulting in the wrong type of analysis being performed on the biopsy samples.

While the doctor did not charge an office fee for the second hole-punch procedure, I <u>was charged</u> for a second lab analysis for the repeated biopsy.

I also remember at one point, being sent by a doctor's office to another city that was 35 miles distance from them, to have blood drawn, due to the office not having an in-house testing lab and not being located in a city, large enough to have a hospital testing lab. Upon our arrival, which was two days later (my wife and I), the lab informed us that the doctor's office had not transmitted the requisition to them. We were required to spend several hours longer at this location, than we had planned, as we waited for the requisition to be faxed from my doctor's office. This required three additional phone-requests by the blood testing lab. The hospital representative who made these calls mentioned to us having to literally demand that they fax the requisition.

This same scenario has occurred at pharmacies we have prescriptions filled at, who have to repeatedly call doctor's offices to get prescriptions transmitted to them, after we have been required to check for these repeatedly over several day periods.

We now ask for written prescriptions, before leaving the doctor's office because there have been some instances in which I could not take my daily thyroid medication dose for several days due to a delay in transmission of electronic prescriptions by doctor's office staff (I now get refills further in advance of running out). Several other members of my family have experienced this same problem, including my mother who takes medications for a heart condition.

After approximately two more years of increasing neuropathy symptoms, I deepened my own online research on possible causes. I began to request tests from my newest doctor that had never been ordered for me, that might reveal the cause of my peripheral neuropathy.

This included a brain MRI, an ultrasound of my liver (this one revealed that I had non-alcoholic fatty liver but no cirrhosis), a thyroid ultrasound (this one further confirmed my diagnosis of Hashimoto's thyroiditis but no cancer or large thyroid nodules were found), blood tests for other autoimmune diseases and my vitamin levels.

The vitamin tests I asked for, revealed that I had vitamin D deficiency and an insufficient level of B12, which my doctor began treatment for via replacement vitamins. These treatments still did not affect improvement for my neuropathy symptoms, after many months and so I asked my doctor's office for a referral to a neurologist. After several weeks of not receiving that requested-referral I eventually resorted to contacting a neurologist directly and they accepted me as a new patient.

The neurologist diagnosed yet another vitamin deficiency I was experiencing via blood testing, this time being a very low level of vitamin E. This finding alone, could explain my development of peripheral neuropathy. I also had abnormal readings on a nerve conduction study that measures the amplitude of signals being conducted by large fiber nerves, further confirming nerve disease. My vitamin deficiencies were further evaluated for a cause of them but it was determined that I did not have a malabsorption syndrome of any type nor do I have cirrhosis of my liver biliary tract, as a cause.

In many cases, nutritional deficiencies can be caused by improper diet or can be idiopathic (no cause determined), the latter apparently being the case with my deficiencies.

My greatest concern regarding my personal diagnoses, as I have just described, is the fact of how often I had to suggest tests or referrals that my doctor should have referred me to or ordered for me directly. While I believe reasonable input should be expected by medical patients, I do not believe they should have to do a doctor's job for them, in the face of obvious steps that need to be taken.

CHAPTER TWO

A Disturbing Statistic Regarding Botched Medical Care

While my personal story of struggles to receive proper diagnostic tests from doctors and proper treatments was somewhat lengthy, I related the information to demonstrate what some patients go through in regard to obtaining proper medical diagnosis and care. I did not relate these incidents, in an attempt to degrade medical doctors or their staff, generally or to cast dispersions of any kind on the medical community. I have the common sense and appreciation, knowing that there are many compassionate doctors, who take proper time and care with their patients and that there are highly efficient medical personnel at doctor's offices and hospitals as well.

With this said, there are also those doctors who are not compassionate, due to various reasons, including a problem medical research groups refer to as "doctor burnout". The staff at these types of doctor's offices often reflect the same attitude of burn out as physicians they work for.

They may also instruct their staff to screen-out (avoid) as much communication and duties as possible, to reduce workload and so that more patients can be fit into the appointments schedules. This method however, when taken too far, can result in inadequate care for patients who attend the appointments of these doctors. While these types of comments are possibly offensive to those who work in the medical field, they are no-less facts and they are problems that cannot be ignored for the sake of not offending someone because the lives of medical patients are at stake.

"Many doctors experience a reality shock at the beginning of their professional careers due to the great discrepancy between expectations and reality. Frustration and overwork eventually develop into exhaustion, often substance misuse and resignation." (The U.S. National Institutes of Health/PubMed – Article titled: "Burnout in doctors")

"It is typically associated with the prolonged and cumulative effects of emotional stress and pressure that arise from personal interaction with members of the public on a daily basis. ---

Where studied, the prevalence amongst healthcare workers approaches 25%." (From the article titled: "Burnout in the Medical Profession" - Egton Medical Information Systems/UK: Dr Tim Kenny, BMedSci (Hons), MB, BS, MRCGP, DCH and Dr Beverley Kenny, MB, BS, MRCGP)

The quotes above, are added to point-out that the problem is also detrimental to doctors and medical staff, whose lives and health are certainly also important. This also demonstrates the fact that this problem is actually a dilemma because doctors can often be terribly overworked as a result of a shortage of them. I believe this to be the case in the state I reside-in (Oklahoma); possibly more-so than in other US states and I have in-fact seen media statistics to this effect, such as the one following.

"...Oklahoma lags on a new state scorecard about health system performance. ...The bottom five states are Nevada, Arkansas, Texas, Mississippi, and Oklahoma." (Source: WebMD – from the article titled: "How States Rank on Health Care" - published in 2007: updated in 2011)

The mishandling of medical care is the 3rd leading cause of death in the US according to The Journal of the American Medical Association (JAMA). Everything possible should be done to lower that statistic and to prevent the problem from becoming even larger. My own daughter was nearly a part of that statistic, when she was in her teens and a busy pharmacy inadvertently gave her a high-dose prescription of a diabetes medication that was intended for an elderly man, instead of being given the acne medication that was prescribed for her. If we had not had the forethought to read the prescription bottle, in addition to the information-insert about the medication that we requested, she would have taken the drug and the effects could have been detrimental at her then petite weight of less than 100lb.

My dad-in-law succumbed to an early death some years ago, after complaining of moderate symptoms that indicated a heart problem after mowing his lawn. He also complained of a tumor on the back of his head. They scheduled him for heart-valve replacement surgery but found a small mass in his lung during x-rays.

They said it was probably scar tissue and to not worry about it or about the tumor on his head. He died within a few months of the surgery, after cancer spread aggressively throughout his body. His children inquired with his health care providers as to why the cancer wasn't further investigated and rather than answer their questions, the hospital cancelled the bill that was owed for his heart surgery. This was admission by the medical entities involved, of improper care but the family did not pursue the issue any further because they knew this would not change the fact of his passing.

My own mother almost died while having a routine colonoscopy procedure. They started the procedure too soon after giving anesthesia and she was screaming; "STOP, I'm still awake"! They gave her more general anesthesia but apparently a dose that was dangerously high and her vital signs dropped to dangerously low levels (respiratory below 60%). A concerned nurse called my dad into her recovery room, to tell him what was happening but after careful monitoring she survived thankfully, despite this potentially fatal error.

The hospital called and apologized only after my mother complained to her regular doctor regarding the error.

My reason for relating these additional stories is to point-out the fact that medical research groups are stating that patients who are "activated" and "self-educated" to a reasonable degree actually receive better care and have better treatment outcomes, than do patients who are not self-advocating and partnering with their doctors (more on this in the next chapter). Medical errors are a major cause of injury and death in the USA each year as previously stated but patients can play a part in helping to avoid some of these errors by offering input to their doctors, in regard to concerns and questions they may have about their symptoms, diagnosis and treatments. As patients, we are in-essence, helping our doctors to do a better job with our medical care, especially in consideration of their extremely busy schedules and most doctors will appreciate this type of partnering, although there can certainly be exceptions, with some doctors wanting minimal to no input from their patients.

When doctor burn out is suspected by a patient or improper handling of patient records by medical staff, patients should seriously consider finding medical care elsewhere if possible (i.e. if insurance and location allows). This is similar in-thought to what is referred to as "second opinions", when a medical diagnosis is in-question and some medical doctors actually recommend them, when diagnoses are of a serious nature or when they involve complicated medical procedures or surgeries.

CHAPTER THREE

What Experts Have to Say about Proactive Patients

Following are two quotes from medical organizations regarding doctor-patient communication:

The National Academy of Medicine:
"Establishing and maintaining strong partnerships between health care providers and patients is crucial to reducing medical errors."

Mack Lipkin MD, founding president of the American Academy on Physician and Patient:
"An activated patient who asks questions and negotiates with the doctor has better outcomes ...The most important predictor of compliance is trust in the doctor; that begins with communication."

These quotes are telling us that proactive, self-educated medical patients have better outcomes and they can improve treatment results by partnering with their doctors, according to the experts.

In regard to the "patients should not research medical issues on your own" idea that we may sometimes see expressed, I would think that most doctors appreciate those patients who reasonably self-educate. I actually had one of my past doctors to tell me that "you can't believe anything you see on the internet"; after I had shown him some pages I copied off the Mayo Clinic and Baptist Hospital websites, regarding my health issues. I had another Dr. actually laugh at me because I researched and listed some things on a sheet to give him at one of my follow-up visits.

The fact is however, that knowledge is vastly important in regard to patient medical issues but even a dozen 10-minite Dr. Office visits will not give one much to go on, unless they are seeing a doctor that actually informs them as thoroughly as they need to be, regarding their medical issues. The fact is that too many patients are needlessly struggling to get better treatment and this is often not accomplished if they do not become involved proactively in their diagnoses and treatments and this includes self-educating to a reasonable degree, through reputable medical sources, whether online or otherwise.

CHAPTER FOUR

How can Patients and Doctors Improve Medical Care?

Smart Preparation for Doctor Visits

With doctor's offices being very busy and sometimes overbooked with ill patients, there are three important steps patients can do to help them achieve optimal results from doctor visits. These will be covered in the subheadings that follow and can help to optimize doctor office visits and to make them as effective for both the doctor and the patient as possible.

Write down your symptoms in detail and any questions you wish to ask your doctor and take the list with you to your office visit.

The reason this step is so important is because it assures that you will leave nothing out of the information that is important for your doctor to know about your illness or health concerns. Office visits at non-specialized doctor offices are roughly timed so that the doctor is in the examining room with each patient for approximately 8 to 10 minutes.

When you have all the information you need to share with him on paper, it can be covered more quickly by simply going down the list, rather than having to stop and remember each thing that might be of significance. When your doctor sees your list in front of you, he or she will most likely have the courtesy to wait for you to express those things you have listed.

Research your illness, to gain some basic knowledge, which will help you communicate better with your doctor.

Most doctors are glad to see that a patient has educated himself generally about the illness or health condition he has as previously mentioned. This saves him from having to give the patient a basic overview or to educate him further about his condition at the time of an office visit. Doing a search on the Internet on health conditions, diseases and illnesses is the single most efficient way to learn information from reliable sources. When doing so however, it is always important to gather the information from reliable, reputable medical sources.

This would include the Mayo Clinic, the Merck Manual Website, the U.S. National Institutes of Health (MedLinePlus), and the National Library of Medicine (PubMed). The quality, more mainstream medical sources will assure that a patient, who learns information about a medical condition he is experiencing, will be getting reliable information to help educate him with general information about symptoms, diagnosis and treatment for his condition.

Take your spouse, friend or relative to your doctor office visit, for support and a second set of ears.

It is a known fact that many patients are nervous when seeing their doctors. Nervousness can be a distraction, making it more difficult for them to comprehend everything the doctor is explaining. Another person accompanying them in the examining room can help to keep them calmer and more focused for concentrating on what their doctor needs to inform them about. The second person a patient takes with them can also serve as a second set of ears, in helping to remember the information being given.

Some patients take micro cassette recorders into the examining room with them, to make sure they have a record of everything the doctor informs them about. This may be a good idea if one does not have a spouse, friend or relative available at the time of an office visit and if it is permissible by the doctor.

All three of these steps can contribute toward improved communication with your doctor and in partnering with him or her, the best possible, to help optimize the results of your treatments.

Doctors Who Listen to Their Patients

The U.S. National Institutes of Health (NIH) and other medical groups are starting to warn about doctor burn-out, as previously mentioned and they are also beginning to educate the public to look for signs of this. An NIH radio ad I have heard recently states that "doctors tend to clam-up" when patients are not communicative with them. One important consideration regarding this problem is in regard to how well a doctor listens to his patient and how well he responds with communication.

Some doctors do not listen well to their patients or they only listen to them selectively, so that they hear only part of what they are saying regarding their health concerns and symptoms. I have actually discontinued with doctors for this very reason, in order to find ones willing to listen and that do not keep me on a strict time-clock.

At the same time, I'm respectful of their time and do not feel that I have ever taken advantage of it. A doctor, who does listen, will have greater success with proper diagnoses and treatments, via ordering proper diagnostic testing and procedures that are determined as being needed by their patients.

Blood Tests

Ask your Doctor to Order Blood Tests

Doctors are not perfect and they cannot feel in your body what you do. They can treat you according to your symptoms but even this requires detailed input by the patient.

If you have come across information online, through reputable medical sources that you feel is significant in regard to your case (i.e. blood tests needing ordered), you need to discuss this with your doctor.

I have been to doctors who were opposed to any input from me as the patient as previously mentioned and they were also opposed to my learning about my illness on fellow patient forums or reputable medical websites, while others have actually appreciated my pro-activeness because it helped them to better optimize my treatment. The NIH radio campaign I mentioned earlier, actually encourages patients to be more informative with their doctors and to ask them questions. The attitude of a doctor in this area may also help you decide whether he is the doctor for you or if you need to seek one who allows more cooperation from you.

Medical blood lab testing is the single most valuable diagnostic testing that is available. Without blood testing, many diseases and disorders, including thyroid hormone disorders would be much more difficult for medical professionals to diagnose.

Understanding your Blood Lab Results

Certainly a patient cannot assume a diagnosis from reading their own blood lab results but this requires a licensed medical professional. They can however learn how to basically interpret them, as to whether a result is normal or abnormal and if outside of normal values, how far outside of the range the result is. Basically understanding blood tests results can help a patient to better discuss them with their doctors.

All lab results have a column beside the title/name of the test that lists your "result" and there will also be a column that lists the "reference range" or "normal values" for each test. When you compare your result to the reference range, this will tell you where your result falls within the normal range or outside of it. Most lab results that fall outside the normal values are "flagged" as abnormal or are highlighted. The lab result page will either have an abnormal column for which to list the flagged results or they will have a notation beside the result such as "L" (meaning low) and "H" (meaning high).

Even results that are within the normal values are not always acceptable as being in a healthy range because with some tests, a borderline high or low level (on the edge of becoming abnormal) indicates the need for close observation and follow-up evaluations. Diseases, such as borderline diabetes and sub-clinical hormone deficiencies for example, are results that usually need to be followed up on (to monitor for possible development of full-blown disease).

If you do not understand what an abnormally high or low result on particular medical tests means, your doctor should help to inform you about them but you may also want to do a search on the Internet using the name of the blood test as the search term. You will find medical lab websites that will inform you as to what an abnormally high or abnormally low result means and many of the major blood testing labs offer this general information online.

Self-Advocating versus Self-Diagnosing

While some people may view this is a form of self-diagnosis or self-treatment, this is not the case.

Doctors are sometimes limited in their time for informing patients thoroughly about their health disorders and patients need a basic understanding of what an abnormal result may mean for them.

Gaining an understanding of a health disorder versus attempting to treat one, are not the same thing. True medical disorders and diseases require professional attention by a licensed physician and patients do not have the ability to obtain treatments that can only be obtained through prescriptions or requisitions provided by medical doctors.

Doctors often have time limited to administering treatments, without passing much information on to the patient about their illness, due to increasing numbers of patients and doctor-shortages. It should be recognized that patients have a right to know what is affecting their lives and health.

Simply gaining some basic understanding about their illness will not take away from the fact that they will still need a licensed physician to treat them and to prescribe the medications needed.

Adequate Mediation by Medical Staff at Hospitals and Doctor's Offices

Medical personnel who are in charge of relaying messages and paperwork, between doctors and patients, should take this responsibility as being extremely serious. I state this, due to the statistics regarding the failure of medical offices, to report, forward and follow-up on abnormal testing results for patients. Following is a quote from "The Center for Advancing Health", who quoted statistics from a medical research study, on their "Health Behavior News Service website".

"In a 2008 study of testing errors, researchers found that nearly three out of four patients involved in a testing error had their treatment delayed, or suffered additional pain, or had a worse health outcome as a result of the error." (From the article titled: "Talking about Medical Tests with Your Health Care Team").

Recently, my brother who is one year older than I, had blood testing ordered, after he began to experience worsening fatigue and a general sense of feeling unwell.

The doctor found that he had diabetes and began treatment for his elevated blood glucose. My brother shared his test results with me, after obtaining copies of them, at my suggestion. I found where he had five different readings flagged low on his blood counts, including his hemoglobin and I suggested that this meant that he also had anemia. He was shocked to hear this due to the fact that no mention of his abnormal readings in the complete blood counts section of his blood test results was ever mentioned to him. His doctor admitted to overlooking these results, at his next office visit with him and the anemia was then treated and monitored, in addition to his diabetes.

It is possible that this was due to medical staff error rather than the doctor being at fault but regardless, these types of errors should not occur and patients should always ask for copies of blood and other medical tests, as a safeguard against abnormal results being overlooked. While a patient cannot self-diagnose, they can point-out any flagged results that are of concern that the doctor has yet to go over with them.

The Relaying of Messages by Medical Workers

When patients call their doctor's offices, to report a concern to their doctors, the receptionists or nurses receiving such messages, should not fail to forward them to the doctor in a timely fashion. In some cases, a patient might be reporting adverse reactions to a medication or a change in their symptoms that the doctor will need to take action regarding. The same is true of messages a doctors asks a staff member to report to a patient. There can be failure for messages to be forwarded and I have heard this scenario related by a number of people in recent years who became upset when their information was not forwarded to the doctor or when information from their doctors, failed to be given to them.

While it is true that doctor's offices can literally be bombarded by incoming messages from patients and that medical workers often try to avoid interrupting a doctor's schedule more often than is necessary, the life and health of patients should not be placed in jeopardy as a result. High priority should be given to the mediation of communication between patients and doctors.

Inadequate staffing should be fixed, if this proves to be a problem because the medical care nurses and office-staff help to provide will otherwise suffer as a consequence. Medical workers should also be protective of a doctor's time within proper perspective and if their job is threatened because they are properly forwarding communication, they should consider reporting this to a medical practices bureau or consider relocating to an office that will better utilize their duties and responsibilities.

In Conclusion:

The medical profession is a God-send in my opinion but there are several different hindrances that can occur, that negatively and seriously affect patients who are treated. I personally feel that the medical profession is a calling and certainly not simply a career-move for those who may enter into it. It is possible that burn out of doctors occurs more often in those who enter the field, without actually seeing it as a calling and who do not see the oath they take when accepting responsibility for the health of others, as seriously as they should.

Certainly this is not true in all cases and there have likely been many sincere, compassionate doctors who have experienced burn out.

While it could be viewed as being wrong for a non medical professional to address the subject that I have covered in the preceding chapters, I would respectfully disagree. I feel my past experiences as I have related them and that I have seen experienced by my family members, qualifies me to address the subject of patient-doctor partnering, from the patient-perspective. It is my sincere hope that I have done so in balance and that nothing contained within the preceding chapters is perceived in any way, as an attack on the medical profession (Thank God for doctors and medical workers). I have expressed these chapters with genuine concern and in hopes that they will inspire my fellow medical patients who read this book, to become proactive in helping their doctors to provide them with best-possible health care.

(END)

About the Author:

I am a husband, father, grandfather and lifetime contract salesman, with experience in health writing that began in 2004. I completed theological studies with Liberty University in 1996. I formerly served as editor and forum moderator of Thyroid Health for a major multi-topic content site and as a general health writer for another, where I received Editor's Choice Awards for my articles on health subjects.

In 2003 I was diagnosed with hypothyroidism; "Hashimoto's thyroiditis" being the cause. This autoimmune form of thyroid disease that causes destruction of the thyroid gland resulted in my also developing "Chronic Fatigue Syndrome", due to a compromised immune system with severe co-morbid "Adrenal Fatigue". I also suffered severe anxiety symptoms, including panic attacks early into the onset of Hashimoto's thyroiditis (Hashitoxicosis). A common heart murmur I was diagnosed with in my teens called "Mitral Valve Prolapse", also worsened in severity of symptoms, with the development of these other health disorders.

My eventual receiving of diagnoses was a difficult process with proper diagnostic testing not being ordered by the first doctors I sought treatment from. These types of issues were inspiration for me to become proactive in my own health care and to self-educate myself on these health disorders, which I have done extensively since 2003. I now enjoy sharing this information with other patients experiencing my same health disorders.

During the early 1990s, I marketed an outdoors product I invented and that I formed a small corporation to patent, manufacture and sell called the "Rod Floater" (now a registered Trademark). I traveled the U.S. making presentations to groups of Wal-Mart zone and district managers and received authorization to sell the product in two regions of Wal-Mart stores for five years.

I also sold the product to Bass Pro Shops, Cabela's and Academy Stores, all of which still carry the product and I landed a national promotion for the product with Kerr-McGee Oil Company who began using the product to promote their outboard motor oil in 1992.

In 1996 I licensed the product to TTI-Blakemore, a major fishing tackle conglomerate, from which I am still paid royalties from sales of the product.

I invented and marketed five additional outdoors products, also getting these into Wal-Mart stores and afterward sold them outright rather than licensing them. I learned a great deal about invention marketing during those years and was privileged to meet the CEOs of many well-known companies. I was also invited for television and radio appearances and met with the T.V. hosts of many fishing shows and was featured in the May 2001 issue of Inventors digest magazine.